This Mediterranean Diet

Journal Belongs To:

BEFORE & After

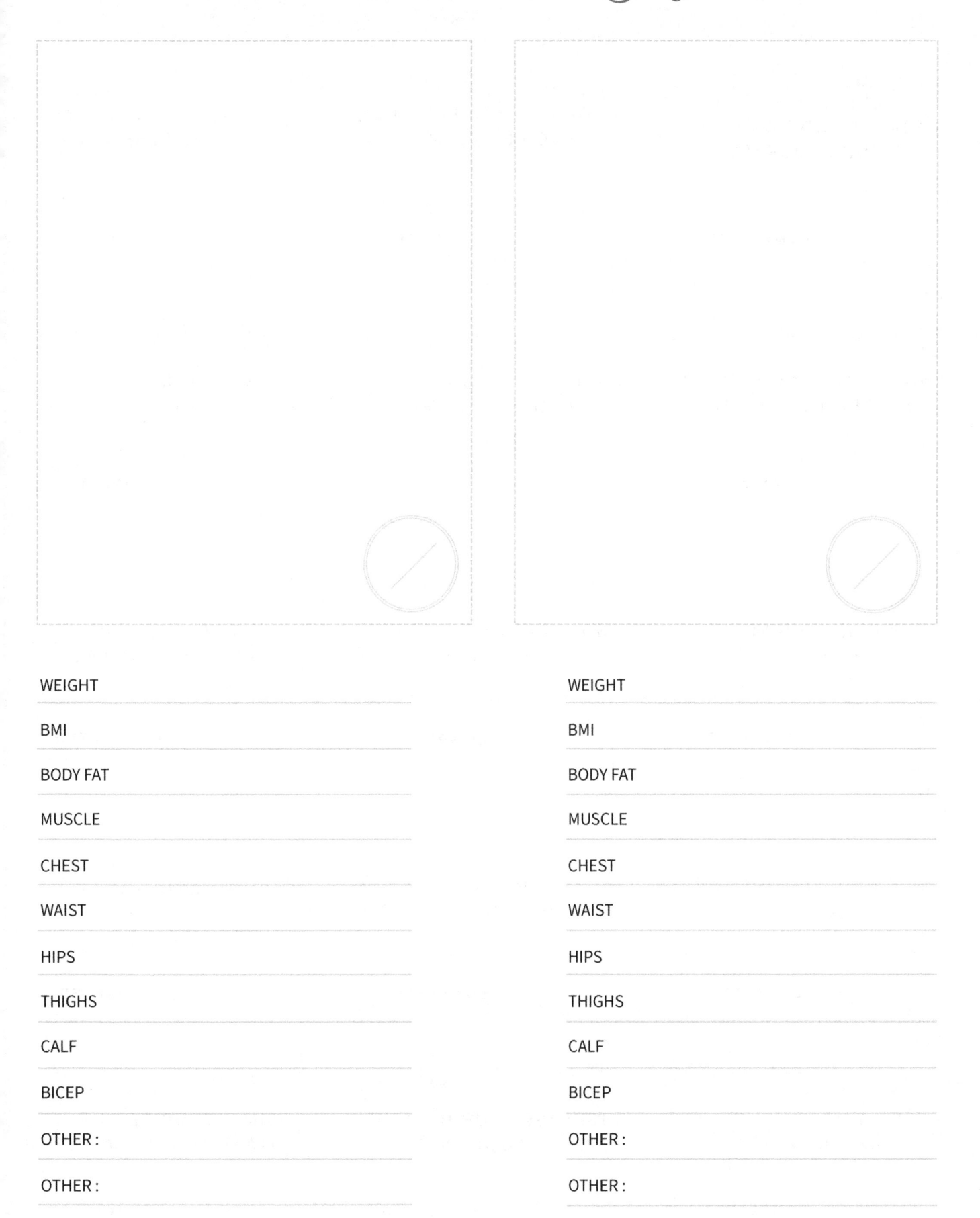

WEIGHT	WEIGHT
BMI	BMI
BODY FAT	BODY FAT
MUSCLE	MUSCLE
CHEST	CHEST
WAIST	WAIST
HIPS	HIPS
THIGHS	THIGHS
CALF	CALF
BICEP	BICEP
OTHER :	OTHER :
OTHER :	OTHER :

Med 15 Task Challenge

1. CREATE A MED JOURNAL AND DOCUMENT YOUR PROGRESS — COMPLETED ☐

2. CHOOSE 7 MED FRIENDLY RECIPES TO TRY — COMPLETED ☐

3. CREATE A WEEKLY MEAL PLANNER — COMPLETED ☐

4. LOG EVERYTHING YOU EAT IN A WEIGHT LOSS APP — COMPLETED ☐

5. PURCHASE A FOOD SCALE AND SPIRALIZER — COMPLETED ☐

6. TRY BULLET PROOF COFFEE — COMPLETED ☐

7. WEIGH YOURSELF EVERY WEEK — COMPLETED ☐

8. GO ALCOHOL FREE FOR ONE WEEK — COMPLETED ☐

9. TRY A 12-HOUR INTERMITTENT FAST — COMPLETED ☐

10. CHECK AND LOG YOUR BODY MEASUREMENTS — COMPLETED ☐

11. LIST ALL THE REASONS WHY MED WILL WORK FOR YOU — COMPLETED ☐

12. LEARN TO DRINK AT LEAST 8 GLASES OF WATER EVERY DAY — COMPLETED ☐

13. MONITOR YOUR WATER INTAKE — COMPLETED ☐

14. INCREASE YOUR HEALTHY PLANT FOOD INTAKE — COMPLETED ☐

15. LIMIT YOUR RED MEAT INTAKE TO ONCE A WEEK — COMPLETED ☐

30 Days of MED

STARTING WEIGHT: **DAY 30 WEIGHT:**

(1) (2) (3) (4) (5) (6) (7) (8) (9) (10)   **LBS LOST:**   **INCHES LOST:**

(11) (12) (13) (14) (15) (16) (17) (18) (19) (20)   **LBS LOST:**   **INCHES LOST:**

(21) (22) (23) (24) (25) (26) (27) (28) (29) (30)   **LBS LOST:**   **INCHES LOST:**

TOTAL WEIGHT LOST: **TOTAL INCHES LOST:**

NOTES:

PERSONAL ACCOMPLISHMENTS:

THOUGHTS & REFLECTIONS:

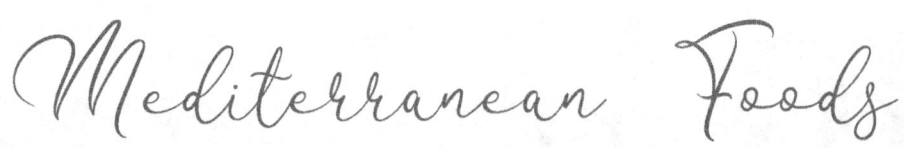

Mediterranean Foods

FISH/SEAFOOD	VEGGIES	VEGGIES	FRUITS
Anchovy	Avocado	Cucumber	Blackberries
Haddock / Cod	Asparagus	Chards	Cranberries
Halibut	Argula	Bell Peppers	Blueberries
Crab/Lobster	Broccoli	Green Beans	Lemon
Mackerel	Cauliflower	Collards	Lime
Salmon	Brussel Sprouts	Mushrooms	Raspberries
Tuna	Cabbage	Spinach	Strawberries
Red Snapper	Celery	Olives	Plantains (paleo)

DAIRY	CONDIMENTS	OILS & FATS	HERBS & SPICES
Cheese (all kinds)	Balsamic Vinegar	Avocado Oil	Garlic
Sour Cream	Beef/Chicken Broth	Butter	Salt & Pepper
Cream Cheese	Bonito Flakes	Coconut Butter	Oregano
Heavy Cream	Tartar Sauce (keto)	Duck Fat	Paprika
Greek Yogurt	Dijon Mustard	Lard/Ghee	Cumin
Almond Milk	Mayo	Nut Oils	Chili Pepper
Cashew Milk	Low Sugar Ketchup	Olive Oil	Basil
Coconut Cream	Pickles	Pork Rinds	Ginger

BAKING	MEATS	DRINKS	MISC.
Almond Flour	Chicken	Diet Soda (moderation)	Canned Tuna
Almond Meal	Beef	Coffee	Pesto
Cashew Flour	Pork	Tea	Soy Sauce
Oat Fiber	Veal	Gatorade Zero	Aioli
Psyllium Husk	Duck	Protein Shake	Béarnaise
Whey Protein	Turkey	Club Soda	Vinaigrette
Flax meal		Broth	Hot Sauce
Hazelnut Flour		Coconut Water	Guacamole

NOTES:

WEIGHT LOSS *Start Date*

Outline your most important fitness goals

Describe how you see yourself in six months

DATE	MED WEIGHT LOSS ACTION PLAN		PERSONAL MILESTONES
		☐	
		☐	
		☐	
		☐	
		☐	
		☐	
		☐	
		☐	
		☐	
		☐	
		☐	
		☐	

Day 1

DATE _____

MY WEIGHT LOSS DIARY:
_____
_____
_____
_____

WATER TRACKER

○ ○ ○ ○ ○ ○ ○ ○

NOTES & REMINDERS

DOODLE MY MOOD

LOW CARB SNACKS

BREAKFAST IDEAS

LUNCH IDEAS

DINNER IDEAS

MY PROGRESS *Tracker* — Day 1

SLEEP TRACKER:

☀ RISE: ___ 🌙 BEDTIME: ___ 💤 SLEEP (HRS): ___

NOTES FOR THE DAY

_____
_____
_____

IN A STATE OF KETOSIS?

YES   NO   UNSURE

WATER INTAKE TRACKER

EXERCISE / WORKOUT ROUTINE

DAILY ENERGY LEVEL

HIGH   MEDIUM   LOW

BREAKFAST

FAT: CARBS: PROTEIN: CALORIES:

LUNCH

FAT: CARBS: PROTEIN: CALORIES:

DINNER

FAT: CARBS: PROTEIN: CALORIES:

SNACKS

FAT: CARBS: PROTEIN: CALORIES:

TOP 6 PRIORITIES OF THE DAY

END OF THE DAY TOTAL OVERVIEW

CARBS   FAT   PROTEIN   CALORIES

Day 2

DATE _____

MY WEIGHT LOSS DIARY:
_____
_____
_____
_____

WATER TRACKER

NOTES & REMINDERS

DOODLE MY MOOD

LOW CARB SNACKS

BREAKFAST IDEAS

LUNCH IDEAS

DINNER IDEAS

MY PROGRESS *Tracker* — Day 2

SLEEP TRACKER:

RISE: _____   BEDTIME: _____   SLEEP (HRS): _____

NOTES FOR THE DAY

_____
_____

IN A STATE OF KETOSIS?

YES   NO   UNSURE

WATER INTAKE TRACKER

EXERCISE / WORKOUT ROUTINE

DAILY ENERGY LEVEL		
HIGH	**MEDIUM**	**LOW**

BREAKFAST

FAT: CARBS: PROTEIN: CALORIES:

LUNCH

FAT: CARBS: PROTEIN: CALORIES:

DINNER

FAT: CARBS: PROTEIN: CALORIES:

SNACKS

FAT: CARBS: PROTEIN: CALORIES:

TOP 6 PRIORITIES OF THE DAY

END OF THE DAY TOTAL OVERVIEW

CARBS   FAT   PROTEIN   CALORIES

Day 3

DATE _____

MY WEIGHT LOSS DIARY:
_____
_____
_____
_____

WATER TRACKER

LOW CARB SNACKS

NOTES & REMINDERS

DOODLE MY MOOD

BREAKFAST IDEAS

LUNCH IDEAS

DINNER IDEAS

MY PROGRESS Tracker — Day 3

SLEEP TRACKER:

RISE: _____   BEDTIME: _____   SLEEP (HRS): _____

NOTES FOR THE DAY

_____
_____
_____

IN A STATE OF KETOSIS?

YES   NO   UNSURE

WATER INTAKE TRACKER

EXERCISE / WORKOUT ROUTINE

DAILY ENERGY LEVEL		
HIGH	MEDIUM	LOW

BREAKFAST

FAT: CARBS: PROTEIN: CALORIES:

LUNCH

FAT: CARBS: PROTEIN: CALORIES:

DINNER

FAT: CARBS: PROTEIN: CALORIES:

SNACKS

FAT: CARBS: PROTEIN: CALORIES:

TOP 6 PRIORITIES OF THE DAY

END OF THE DAY TOTAL OVERVIEW

CARBS   FAT   PROTEIN   CALORIES

Day 4

DATE _____

MY WEIGHT LOSS DIARY:
_____
_____
_____
_____

WATER TRACKER

NOTES & REMINDERS

DOODLE MY MOOD

LOW CARB SNACKS

BREAKFAST IDEAS

LUNCH IDEAS

DINNER IDEAS

MY PROGRESS *Tracker* — Day 4

SLEEP TRACKER:

RISE: _____   BEDTIME: _____   SLEEP (HRS): _____

NOTES FOR THE DAY

_____
_____
_____

IN A STATE OF KETOSIS?

YES   NO   UNSURE

WATER INTAKE TRACKER

EXERCISE / WORKOUT ROUTINE

DAILY ENERGY LEVEL

| HIGH | MEDIUM | LOW |

BREAKFAST

FAT: CARBS: PROTEIN: CALORIES:

LUNCH

FAT: CARBS: PROTEIN: CALORIES:

DINNER

FAT: CARBS: PROTEIN: CALORIES:

SNACKS

FAT: CARBS: PROTEIN: CALORIES:

TOP 6 PRIORITIES OF THE DAY

END OF THE DAY TOTAL OVERVIEW

CARBS   FAT   PROTEIN   CALORIES

Day 5

DATE _____

MY WEIGHT LOSS DIARY:
_____
_____
_____
_____

WATER TRACKER

NOTES & REMINDERS

DOODLE MY MOOD

LOW CARB SNACKS

BREAKFAST IDEAS

LUNCH IDEAS

DINNER IDEAS

MY PROGRESS *Tracker* — Day 5

SLEEP TRACKER:

RISE: _____   BEDTIME: _____   SLEEP (HRS): _____

NOTES FOR THE DAY

_____
_____
_____

IN A STATE OF KETOSIS?

YES   NO   UNSURE

WATER INTAKE TRACKER

EXERCISE / WORKOUT ROUTINE

DAILY ENERGY LEVEL

| HIGH | MEDIUM | LOW |

BREAKFAST
FAT: CARBS: PROTEIN: CALORIES:

LUNCH
FAT: CARBS: PROTEIN: CALORIES:

DINNER
FAT: CARBS: PROTEIN: CALORIES:

SNACKS
FAT: CARBS: PROTEIN: CALORIES:

TOP 6 PRIORITIES OF THE DAY

END OF THE DAY TOTAL OVERVIEW

CARBS   FAT   PROTEIN   CALORIES

Day 6

DATE _____

MY WEIGHT LOSS DIARY:
_____
_____
_____
_____

WATER TRACKER

NOTES & REMINDERS

DOODLE MY MOOD

LOW CARB SNACKS

BREAKFAST IDEAS

LUNCH IDEAS

DINNER IDEAS

MY PROGRESS *Tracker* — Day 6

SLEEP TRACKER:

☀ RISE: ☾ BEDTIME: 💭 SLEEP (HRS):

NOTES FOR THE DAY

_____
_____
_____

EXERCISE / WORKOUT ROUTINE

TOP 6 PRIORITIES OF THE DAY

IN A STATE OF KETOSIS?

YES   NO   UNSURE

WATER INTAKE TRACKER

DAILY ENERGY LEVEL		
HIGH	**MEDIUM**	**LOW**

BREAKFAST
FAT: CARBS: PROTEIN: CALORIES:

LUNCH
FAT: CARBS: PROTEIN: CALORIES:

DINNER
FAT: CARBS: PROTEIN: CALORIES:

SNACKS
FAT: CARBS: PROTEIN: CALORIES:

END OF THE DAY TOTAL OVERVIEW

CARBS   FAT   PROTEIN   CALORIES

Day 7

DATE _____

MY WEIGHT LOSS DIARY:

_____
_____
_____
_____

WATER TRACKER

NOTES & REMINDERS

DOODLE MY MOOD

LOW CARB SNACKS

BREAKFAST IDEAS

LUNCH IDEAS

DINNER IDEAS

MY PROGRESS Tracker — Day 7

SLEEP TRACKER:

RISE: _____   BEDTIME: _____   SLEEP (HRS): _____

NOTES FOR THE DAY

_____
_____

IN A STATE OF KETOSIS?

YES   NO   UNSURE

WATER INTAKE TRACKER

EXERCISE / WORKOUT ROUTINE

DAILY ENERGY LEVEL

HIGH   MEDIUM   LOW

BREAKFAST

FAT: CARBS: PROTEIN: CALORIES:

LUNCH

FAT: CARBS: PROTEIN: CALORIES:

DINNER

FAT: CARBS: PROTEIN: CALORIES:

SNACKS

FAT: CARBS: PROTEIN: CALORIES:

TOP 6 PRIORITIES OF THE DAY

END OF THE DAY TOTAL OVERVIEW

CARBS   FAT   PROTEIN   CALORIES

Day 8

DATE _____

MY WEIGHT LOSS DIARY:

_____
_____
_____
_____

WATER TRACKER

LOW CARB SNACKS

NOTES & REMINDERS

DOODLE MY MOOD

BREAKFAST IDEAS

LUNCH IDEAS

DINNER IDEAS

MY PROGRESS *Tracker* — Day 8

SLEEP TRACKER:

☀️ RISE: ___   🌙 BEDTIME: ___   💭 SLEEP (HRS): ___

NOTES FOR THE DAY

_____
_____
_____

IN A STATE OF KETOSIS?

YES   NO   UNSURE

WATER INTAKE TRACKER

EXERCISE / WORKOUT ROUTINE

DAILY ENERGY LEVEL

| HIGH | MEDIUM | LOW |

BREAKFAST

FAT: CARBS: PROTEIN: CALORIES:

LUNCH

FAT: CARBS: PROTEIN: CALORIES:

DINNER

FAT: CARBS: PROTEIN: CALORIES:

SNACKS

FAT: CARBS: PROTEIN: CALORIES:

TOP 6 PRIORITIES OF THE DAY

END OF THE DAY TOTAL OVERVIEW

CARBS   FAT   PROTEIN   CALORIES

Day 9

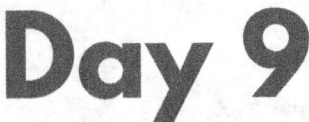

DATE _____

MY WEIGHT LOSS DIARY:
_____
_____
_____
_____

WATER TRACKER

NOTES & REMINDERS

DOODLE MY MOOD

LOW CARB SNACKS

BREAKFAST IDEAS

LUNCH IDEAS

DINNER IDEAS

MY PROGRESS *Tracker* — Day 9

SLEEP TRACKER:

RISE: ___   BEDTIME: ___   SLEEP (HRS): ___

NOTES FOR THE DAY

_____
_____
_____

IN A STATE OF KETOSIS?

YES   NO   UNSURE

WATER INTAKE TRACKER

EXERCISE / WORKOUT ROUTINE

DAILY ENERGY LEVEL

| HIGH | MEDIUM | LOW |

BREAKFAST

FAT: CARBS: PROTEIN: CALORIES:

LUNCH

FAT: CARBS: PROTEIN: CALORIES:

DINNER

FAT: CARBS: PROTEIN: CALORIES:

SNACKS

FAT: CARBS: PROTEIN: CALORIES:

TOP 6 PRIORITIES OF THE DAY

END OF THE DAY TOTAL OVERVIEW

CARBS   FAT   PROTEIN   CALORIES

Day 10

DATE _____

MY WEIGHT LOSS DIARY:

WATER TRACKER

LOW CARB SNACKS

NOTES & REMINDERS

DOODLE MY MOOD

BREAKFAST IDEAS

LUNCH IDEAS

DINNER IDEAS

MY PROGRESS Tracker

Day 10

SLEEP TRACKER:

RISE: _____ BEDTIME: _____ SLEEP (HRS): _____

NOTES FOR THE DAY

_____
_____
_____

IN A STATE OF KETOSIS?

YES   NO   UNSURE

WATER INTAKE TRACKER

EXERCISE / WORKOUT ROUTINE

DAILY ENERGY LEVEL

| HIGH | MEDIUM | LOW |

BREAKFAST
FAT: CARBS: PROTEIN: CALORIES:

LUNCH
FAT: CARBS: PROTEIN: CALORIES:

DINNER
FAT: CARBS: PROTEIN: CALORIES:

SNACKS
FAT: CARBS: PROTEIN: CALORIES:

TOP 6 PRIORITIES OF THE DAY

END OF THE DAY TOTAL OVERVIEW

CARBS   FAT   PROTEIN   CALORIES

Day 11

DATE _____

MY WEIGHT LOSS DIARY:
_____
_____
_____
_____

WATER TRACKER

NOTES & REMINDERS

DOODLE MY MOOD

LOW CARB SNACKS

BREAKFAST IDEAS

LUNCH IDEAS

DINNER IDEAS

MY PROGRESS *Tracker*   **Day 11**

SLEEP TRACKER:

RISE: BEDTIME: SLEEP (HRS):

NOTES FOR THE DAY

_____

_____

_____

IN A STATE OF KETOSIS?

YES   NO   UNSURE

WATER INTAKE TRACKER

EXERCISE / WORKOUT ROUTINE

DAILY ENERGY LEVEL		
HIGH	**MEDIUM**	**LOW**

BREAKFAST
FAT: CARBS: PROTEIN: CALORIES:

LUNCH
FAT: CARBS: PROTEIN: CALORIES:

DINNER
FAT: CARBS: PROTEIN: CALORIES:

SNACKS
FAT: CARBS: PROTEIN: CALORIES:

TOP 6 PRIORITIES OF THE DAY

END OF THE DAY TOTAL OVERVIEW

CARBS   FAT   PROTEIN   CALORIES

Day 12

DATE _____

MY WEIGHT LOSS DIARY:

_____
_____
_____
_____

WATER TRACKER	NOTES & REMINDERS	DOODLE MY MOOD

LOW CARB SNACKS

BREAKFAST IDEAS | **LUNCH IDEAS** | **DINNER IDEAS**

MY PROGRESS *Tracker*   Day 12

SLEEP TRACKER:

☼ RISE: _____   BEDTIME: _____   SLEEP (HRS): _____

NOTES FOR THE DAY

_____
_____
_____

EXERCISE / WORKOUT ROUTINE

TOP 6 PRIORITIES OF THE DAY

○ _____   ○ _____
○ _____   ○ _____
○ _____   ○ _____

IN A STATE OF KETOSIS?

YES   NO   UNSURE

WATER INTAKE TRACKER

DAILY ENERGY LEVEL

HIGH   MEDIUM   LOW

BREAKFAST

FAT: CARBS: PROTEIN: CALORIES:

LUNCH

FAT: CARBS: PROTEIN: CALORIES:

DINNER

FAT: CARBS: PROTEIN: CALORIES:

SNACKS

FAT: CARBS: PROTEIN: CALORIES:

END OF THE DAY TOTAL OVERVIEW

CARBS   FAT   PROTEIN   CALORIES

Day 13

DATE _____

MY WEIGHT LOSS DIARY:
_____
_____
_____
_____

WATER TRACKER
○ ○ ○ ○ ○ ○ ○

LOW CARB SNACKS

NOTES & REMINDERS
_____
_____
_____
_____
_____
_____
_____
_____

DOODLE MY MOOD

BREAKFAST IDEAS

LUNCH IDEAS

DINNER IDEAS

MY PROGRESS Tracker

Day 13

SLEEP TRACKER:

RISE: BEDTIME: SLEEP (HRS):

NOTES FOR THE DAY

IN A STATE OF KETOSIS?

YES   NO   UNSURE

WATER INTAKE TRACKER

EXERCISE / WORKOUT ROUTINE

DAILY ENERGY LEVEL

HIGH   MEDIUM   LOW

BREAKFAST

FAT: CARBS: PROTEIN: CALORIES:

LUNCH

FAT: CARBS: PROTEIN: CALORIES:

DINNER

FAT: CARBS: PROTEIN: CALORIES:

SNACKS

FAT: CARBS: PROTEIN: CALORIES:

TOP 6 PRIORITIES OF THE DAY

END OF THE DAY TOTAL OVERVIEW

CARBS   FAT   PROTEIN   CALORIES

Day 14

DATE _____

MY WEIGHT LOSS DIARY:
_____
_____
_____
_____

WATER TRACKER

LOW CARB SNACKS

NOTES & REMINDERS

DOODLE MY MOOD

BREAKFAST IDEAS

LUNCH IDEAS

DINNER IDEAS

MY PROGRESS *Tracker*   **Day 14**

SLEEP TRACKER:

☀ RISE: 🌙 BEDTIME: 💭 SLEEP (HRS):

NOTES FOR THE DAY

IN A STATE OF KETOSIS?

YES   NO   UNSURE

WATER INTAKE TRACKER

EXERCISE / WORKOUT ROUTINE

DAILY ENERGY LEVEL		
HIGH	**MEDIUM**	**LOW**

BREAKFAST

FAT: CARBS: PROTEIN: CALORIES:

LUNCH

FAT: CARBS: PROTEIN: CALORIES:

DINNER

FAT: CARBS: PROTEIN: CALORIES:

SNACKS

FAT: CARBS: PROTEIN: CALORIES:

TOP 6 PRIORITIES OF THE DAY

END OF THE DAY TOTAL OVERVIEW

CARBS   FAT   PROTEIN   CALORIES

Day 15

DATE _____

MY WEIGHT LOSS DIARY:
_____
_____
_____
_____

WATER TRACKER

NOTES & REMINDERS

DOODLE MY MOOD

LOW CARB SNACKS

BREAKFAST IDEAS

LUNCH IDEAS

DINNER IDEAS

MY PROGRESS Tracker

Day 15

SLEEP TRACKER:

RISE: BEDTIME: SLEEP (HRS):

NOTES FOR THE DAY

IN A STATE OF KETOSIS?

YES   NO   UNSURE

WATER INTAKE TRACKER

EXERCISE / WORKOUT ROUTINE

DAILY ENERGY LEVEL

HIGH   MEDIUM   LOW

BREAKFAST

FAT: CARBS: PROTEIN: CALORIES:

LUNCH

FAT: CARBS: PROTEIN: CALORIES:

DINNER

FAT: CARBS: PROTEIN: CALORIES:

SNACKS

FAT: CARBS: PROTEIN: CALORIES:

TOP 6 PRIORITIES OF THE DAY

END OF THE DAY TOTAL OVERVIEW

CARBS   FAT   PROTEIN   CALORIES

Day 16

DATE _____

MY WEIGHT LOSS DIARY:
_____
_____
_____
_____

WATER TRACKER

NOTES & REMINDERS

DOODLE MY MOOD

LOW CARB SNACKS

BREAKFAST IDEAS

LUNCH IDEAS

DINNER IDEAS

MY PROGRESS Tracker

Day 16

SLEEP TRACKER:

RISE: BEDTIME: SLEEP (HRS):

NOTES FOR THE DAY

IN A STATE OF KETOSIS?

YES   NO   UNSURE

WATER INTAKE TRACKER

EXERCISE / WORKOUT ROUTINE

DAILY ENERGY LEVEL		
HIGH	MEDIUM	LOW

BREAKFAST

FAT: CARBS: PROTEIN: CALORIES:

LUNCH

FAT: CARBS: PROTEIN: CALORIES:

DINNER

FAT: CARBS: PROTEIN: CALORIES:

SNACKS

FAT: CARBS: PROTEIN: CALORIES:

TOP 6 PRIORITIES OF THE DAY

END OF THE DAY TOTAL OVERVIEW

CARBS   FAT   PROTEIN   CALORIES

Day 17

DATE _____

MY WEIGHT LOSS DIARY:
_____
_____
_____
_____

WATER TRACKER

NOTES & REMINDERS

DOODLE MY MOOD

LOW CARB SNACKS

BREAKFAST IDEAS

LUNCH IDEAS

DINNER IDEAS

MY PROGRESS *Tracker*   Day 17

SLEEP TRACKER:

☀ RISE: 🌙 BEDTIME: 💭 SLEEP (HRS):

NOTES FOR THE DAY

_____
_____
_____

EXERCISE / WORKOUT ROUTINE

TOP 6 PRIORITIES OF THE DAY

IN A STATE OF KETOSIS?

YES   NO   UNSURE

WATER INTAKE TRACKER

DAILY ENERGY LEVEL

HIGH	MEDIUM	LOW

BREAKFAST

FAT: CARBS: PROTEIN: CALORIES:

LUNCH

FAT: CARBS: PROTEIN: CALORIES:

DINNER

FAT: CARBS: PROTEIN: CALORIES:

SNACKS

FAT: CARBS: PROTEIN: CALORIES:

END OF THE DAY TOTAL OVERVIEW

CARBS   FAT   PROTEIN   CALORIES

Day 18

DATE _____

MY WEIGHT LOSS DIARY:

WATER TRACKER

NOTES & REMINDERS

DOODLE MY MOOD

LOW CARB SNACKS

BREAKFAST IDEAS

LUNCH IDEAS

DINNER IDEAS

MY PROGRESS *Tracker* — Day 18

SLEEP TRACKER:

RISE: ___ BEDTIME: ___ SLEEP (HRS): ___

NOTES FOR THE DAY

_____
_____
_____

IN A STATE OF KETOSIS?

YES   NO   UNSURE

WATER INTAKE TRACKER

EXERCISE / WORKOUT ROUTINE

DAILY ENERGY LEVEL		
HIGH	MEDIUM	LOW

BREAKFAST

FAT: CARBS: PROTEIN: CALORIES:

LUNCH

FAT: CARBS: PROTEIN: CALORIES:

DINNER

FAT: CARBS: PROTEIN: CALORIES:

SNACKS

FAT: CARBS: PROTEIN: CALORIES:

TOP 6 PRIORITIES OF THE DAY

END OF THE DAY TOTAL OVERVIEW

CARBS   FAT   PROTEIN   CALORIES

Day 19

DATE _____

MY WEIGHT LOSS DIARY:

_____
_____
_____
_____

WATER TRACKER

○ ○ ○ ○ ○ ○ ○

NOTES & REMINDERS

DOODLE MY MOOD

LOW CARB SNACKS

BREAKFAST IDEAS

LUNCH IDEAS

DINNER IDEAS

MY PROGRESS Tracker

Day 19

SLEEP TRACKER:

RISE: BEDTIME: SLEEP (HRS):

NOTES FOR THE DAY

_____
_____
_____

EXERCISE / WORKOUT ROUTINE

TOP 6 PRIORITIES OF THE DAY

IN A STATE OF KETOSIS?

YES   NO   UNSURE

WATER INTAKE TRACKER

DAILY ENERGY LEVEL

HIGH	MEDIUM	LOW

BREAKFAST

FAT: CARBS: PROTEIN: CALORIES:

LUNCH

FAT: CARBS: PROTEIN: CALORIES:

DINNER

FAT: CARBS: PROTEIN: CALORIES:

SNACKS

FAT: CARBS: PROTEIN: CALORIES:

END OF THE DAY TOTAL OVERVIEW

CARBS   FAT   PROTEIN   CALORIES

Day 20

DATE _____

MY WEIGHT LOSS DIARY:
_____
_____
_____
_____

WATER TRACKER

LOW CARB SNACKS

NOTES & REMINDERS

DOODLE MY MOOD

BREAKFAST IDEAS

LUNCH IDEAS

DINNER IDEAS

MY PROGRESS *Tracker* — Day 20

SLEEP TRACKER:

RISE: _____   BEDTIME: _____   SLEEP (HRS): _____

NOTES FOR THE DAY

_____
_____
_____

IN A STATE OF KETOSIS?

YES   NO   UNSURE

WATER INTAKE TRACKER

EXERCISE / WORKOUT ROUTINE

DAILY ENERGY LEVEL

| HIGH | MEDIUM | LOW |

BREAKFAST

FAT: CARBS: PROTEIN: CALORIES:

LUNCH

FAT: CARBS: PROTEIN: CALORIES:

DINNER

FAT: CARBS: PROTEIN: CALORIES:

SNACKS

FAT: CARBS: PROTEIN: CALORIES:

TOP 6 PRIORITIES OF THE DAY

END OF THE DAY TOTAL OVERVIEW

CARBS   FAT   PROTEIN   CALORIES

Day 21

DATE _____

MY WEIGHT LOSS DIARY:
_____
_____
_____
_____

WATER TRACKER

○ ○ ○ ○ ○ ○ ○

LOW CARB SNACKS

NOTES & REMINDERS

DOODLE MY MOOD

BREAKFAST IDEAS

LUNCH IDEAS

DINNER IDEAS

MY PROGRESS *Tracker* — Day 21

SLEEP TRACKER:

RISE: | BEDTIME: | SLEEP (HRS):

NOTES FOR THE DAY

IN A STATE OF KETOSIS?

YES   NO   UNSURE

WATER INTAKE TRACKER

EXERCISE / WORKOUT ROUTINE

DAILY ENERGY LEVEL

HIGH	MEDIUM	LOW

BREAKFAST

FAT: CARBS: PROTEIN: CALORIES:

LUNCH

FAT: CARBS: PROTEIN: CALORIES:

DINNER

FAT: CARBS: PROTEIN: CALORIES:

SNACKS

FAT: CARBS: PROTEIN: CALORIES:

TOP 6 PRIORITIES OF THE DAY

END OF THE DAY TOTAL OVERVIEW

CARBS	FAT	PROTEIN	CALORIES

Day 22

DATE _____

MY WEIGHT LOSS DIARY:
_____
_____
_____
_____

WATER TRACKER

LOW CARB SNACKS

NOTES & REMINDERS

DOODLE MY MOOD

BREAKFAST IDEAS

LUNCH IDEAS

DINNER IDEAS

MY PROGRESS *Tracker* — Day 22

SLEEP TRACKER:

RISE: BEDTIME: SLEEP (HRS):

NOTES FOR THE DAY

IN A STATE OF KETOSIS?

YES   NO   UNSURE

WATER INTAKE TRACKER

EXERCISE / WORKOUT ROUTINE

DAILY ENERGY LEVEL		
HIGH	MEDIUM	LOW

BREAKFAST

FAT: CARBS: PROTEIN: CALORIES:

LUNCH

FAT: CARBS: PROTEIN: CALORIES:

DINNER

FAT: CARBS: PROTEIN: CALORIES:

SNACKS

FAT: CARBS: PROTEIN: CALORIES:

TOP 6 PRIORITIES OF THE DAY

END OF THE DAY TOTAL OVERVIEW

CARBS   FAT   PROTEIN   CALORIES

Day 23

DATE _____

MY WEIGHT LOSS DIARY:
_____
_____
_____
_____

WATER TRACKER

NOTES & REMINDERS

DOODLE MY MOOD

LOW CARB SNACKS

BREAKFAST IDEAS

LUNCH IDEAS

DINNER IDEAS

MY PROGRESS *Tracker*   **Day 23**

SLEEP TRACKER:

RISE: BEDTIME: SLEEP (HRS):

NOTES FOR THE DAY

_____

_____

_____

IN A STATE OF KETOSIS?

YES   NO   UNSURE

WATER INTAKE TRACKER

EXERCISE / WORKOUT ROUTINE

DAILY ENERGY LEVEL
HIGH   **MEDIUM**   **LOW**

BREAKFAST

FAT: CARBS: PROTEIN: CALORIES:

LUNCH

FAT: CARBS: PROTEIN: CALORIES:

DINNER

FAT: CARBS: PROTEIN: CALORIES:

SNACKS

FAT: CARBS: PROTEIN: CALORIES:

TOP 6 PRIORITIES OF THE DAY

END OF THE DAY TOTAL OVERVIEW

CARBS   FAT   PROTEIN   CALORIES

Day 24

DATE _____

MY WEIGHT LOSS DIARY:
_____
_____
_____
_____
_____

WATER TRACKER

LOW CARB SNACKS

NOTES & REMINDERS

DOODLE MY MOOD

BREAKFAST IDEAS

LUNCH IDEAS

DINNER IDEAS

MY PROGRESS *Tracker* — Day 24

SLEEP TRACKER:

RISE: ____ BEDTIME: ____ SLEEP (HRS): ____

NOTES FOR THE DAY

_____
_____
_____

EXERCISE / WORKOUT ROUTINE

TOP 6 PRIORITIES OF THE DAY

IN A STATE OF KETOSIS?

YES   NO   UNSURE

WATER INTAKE TRACKER

DAILY ENERGY LEVEL		
HIGH	**MEDIUM**	**LOW**

BREAKFAST
FAT: CARBS: PROTEIN: CALORIES:

LUNCH
FAT: CARBS: PROTEIN: CALORIES:

DINNER
FAT: CARBS: PROTEIN: CALORIES:

SNACKS
FAT: CARBS: PROTEIN: CALORIES:

END OF THE DAY TOTAL OVERVIEW

CARBS   FAT   PROTEIN   CALORIES

Day 25

DATE _____

MY WEIGHT LOSS DIARY:

_____
_____
_____
_____

WATER TRACKER

NOTES & REMINDERS

DOODLE MY MOOD

LOW CARB SNACKS

BREAKFAST IDEAS

LUNCH IDEAS

DINNER IDEAS

MY PROGRESS *Tracker* — Day 25

SLEEP TRACKER:

☀ RISE: ☾ BEDTIME: 💭 SLEEP (HRS):

NOTES FOR THE DAY

EXERCISE / WORKOUT ROUTINE

TOP 6 PRIORITIES OF THE DAY

IN A STATE OF KETOSIS?

YES   NO   UNSURE

WATER INTAKE TRACKER

DAILY ENERGY LEVEL		
HIGH	MEDIUM	LOW

BREAKFAST

FAT: CARBS: PROTEIN: CALORIES:

LUNCH

FAT: CARBS: PROTEIN: CALORIES:

DINNER

FAT: CARBS: PROTEIN: CALORIES:

SNACKS

FAT: CARBS: PROTEIN: CALORIES:

END OF THE DAY TOTAL OVERVIEW

CARBS   FAT   PROTEIN   CALORIES

Day 26

DATE _____

MY WEIGHT LOSS DIARY:

WATER TRACKER

LOW CARB SNACKS

NOTES & REMINDERS

DOODLE MY MOOD

BREAKFAST IDEAS

LUNCH IDEAS

DINNER IDEAS

MY PROGRESS *Tracker* — Day 26

SLEEP TRACKER:

☀ RISE: 🌙 BEDTIME: 💭 SLEEP (HRS):

NOTES FOR THE DAY

IN A STATE OF KETOSIS?

YES   NO   UNSURE

WATER INTAKE TRACKER

EXERCISE / WORKOUT ROUTINE

DAILY ENERGY LEVEL

HIGH   MEDIUM   LOW

BREAKFAST

FAT: CARBS: PROTEIN: CALORIES:

LUNCH

FAT: CARBS: PROTEIN: CALORIES:

DINNER

FAT: CARBS: PROTEIN: CALORIES:

SNACKS

FAT: CARBS: PROTEIN: CALORIES:

TOP 6 PRIORITIES OF THE DAY

END OF THE DAY TOTAL OVERVIEW

CARBS   FAT   PROTEIN   CALORIES

Day 27

DATE _____

MY WEIGHT LOSS DIARY:
_____
_____
_____
_____

WATER TRACKER

NOTES & REMINDERS

DOODLE MY MOOD

LOW CARB SNACKS

BREAKFAST IDEAS

LUNCH IDEAS

DINNER IDEAS

MY PROGRESS *Tracker* — Day 27

SLEEP TRACKER:

RISE: ___   BEDTIME: ___   SLEEP (HRS): ___

NOTES FOR THE DAY

_____
_____
_____

EXERCISE / WORKOUT ROUTINE

TOP 6 PRIORITIES OF THE DAY

IN A STATE OF KETOSIS?

YES   NO   UNSURE

WATER INTAKE TRACKER

DAILY ENERGY LEVEL
HIGH   MEDIUM   LOW

BREAKFAST
FAT: CARBS: PROTEIN: CALORIES:

LUNCH
FAT: CARBS: PROTEIN: CALORIES:

DINNER
FAT: CARBS: PROTEIN: CALORIES:

SNACKS
FAT: CARBS: PROTEIN: CALORIES:

END OF THE DAY TOTAL OVERVIEW

CARBS   FAT   PROTEIN   CALORIES

Day 28

DATE _____

MY WEIGHT LOSS DIARY:
_____
_____
_____
_____

WATER TRACKER

LOW CARB SNACKS

NOTES & REMINDERS

DOODLE MY MOOD

BREAKFAST IDEAS

LUNCH IDEAS

DINNER IDEAS

MY PROGRESS *Tracker* — Day 28

SLEEP TRACKER:

☼ RISE: ☾ BEDTIME: 💭 SLEEP (HRS):

NOTES FOR THE DAY

_____
_____
_____

IN A STATE OF KETOSIS?

YES   NO   UNSURE

WATER INTAKE TRACKER

EXERCISE / WORKOUT ROUTINE

DAILY ENERGY LEVEL

| HIGH | MEDIUM | LOW |

BREAKFAST

FAT: CARBS: PROTEIN: CALORIES:

LUNCH

FAT: CARBS: PROTEIN: CALORIES:

DINNER

FAT: CARBS: PROTEIN: CALORIES:

SNACKS

FAT: CARBS: PROTEIN: CALORIES:

TOP 6 PRIORITIES OF THE DAY

END OF THE DAY TOTAL OVERVIEW

CARBS   FAT   PROTEIN   CALORIES

Day 29

DATE _____

MY WEIGHT LOSS DIARY:

WATER TRACKER

LOW CARB SNACKS

NOTES & REMINDERS

DOODLE MY MOOD

BREAKFAST IDEAS

LUNCH IDEAS

DINNER IDEAS

MY PROGRESS *Tracker* — Day 29

SLEEP TRACKER:

RISE: ___   BEDTIME: ___   SLEEP (HRS): ___

NOTES FOR THE DAY

_____
_____
_____

IN A STATE OF KETOSIS?

YES   NO   UNSURE

WATER INTAKE TRACKER

EXERCISE / WORKOUT ROUTINE

DAILY ENERGY LEVEL
HIGH   MEDIUM   LOW

BREAKFAST

FAT: CARBS: PROTEIN: CALORIES:

LUNCH

FAT: CARBS: PROTEIN: CALORIES:

DINNER

FAT: CARBS: PROTEIN: CALORIES:

SNACKS

FAT: CARBS: PROTEIN: CALORIES:

TOP 6 PRIORITIES OF THE DAY

END OF THE DAY TOTAL OVERVIEW

CARBS   FAT   PROTEIN   CALORIES

Day 30

DATE _____

MY WEIGHT LOSS DIARY:

_____
_____
_____
_____

WATER TRACKER

NOTES & REMINDERS

DOODLE MY MOOD

LOW CARB SNACKS

BREAKFAST IDEAS

LUNCH IDEAS

DINNER IDEAS

MY PROGRESS *Tracker* — Day 30

SLEEP TRACKER:

RISE: BEDTIME: SLEEP (HRS):

NOTES FOR THE DAY

IN A STATE OF KETOSIS?

YES   NO   UNSURE

WATER INTAKE TRACKER

EXERCISE / WORKOUT ROUTINE

DAILY ENERGY LEVEL

HIGH   **MEDIUM**   **LOW**

BREAKFAST

FAT: CARBS: PROTEIN: CALORIES:

LUNCH

FAT: CARBS: PROTEIN: CALORIES:

DINNER

FAT: CARBS: PROTEIN: CALORIES:

SNACKS

FAT: CARBS: PROTEIN: CALORIES:

TOP 6 PRIORITIES OF THE DAY

END OF THE DAY TOTAL OVERVIEW

CARBS   FAT   PROTEIN   CALORIES

WEIGHT LOSS *Tracker*

WEEKLY WEIGHT LOSS TRACKER

Week 1

DATE: _____ _____ _____ _____ _____ _____

- BUST
- WAIST
- HIPS
- BICEP
- THIGH
- CALF
- WEIGHT

TOTAL WEIGHT LOSS >>

WEIGHT LOSS *Tracker*

WEEKLY WEIGHT LOSS TRACKER

Week 2

DATE:

BUST					
WAIST					
HIPS					
BICEP					
THIGH					
CALF					
WEIGHT					
TOTAL WEIGHT LOSS >>					

WEIGHT LOSS *Tracker*

WEEKLY WEIGHT LOSS TRACKER

Week 3

DATE: _____ _____ _____ _____ _____

	BUST					
	WAIST					
	HIPS					
	BICEP					
	THIGH					
	CALF					
	WEIGHT					
TOTAL WEIGHT LOSS >>						

WEIGHT LOSS *Tracker*

WEEKLY WEIGHT LOSS TRACKER

Week 4

DATE:

BUST					
WAIST					
HIPS					
BICEP					
THIGH					
CALF					
WEIGHT					
TOTAL WEIGHT LOSS >>					

Weekly Meal Planner

Week 1

	Breakfast	Lunch	Dinner	Snack	Other
Monday	Carbs Fat Protein Cals TOTAL	Carbs Fat Protein Cals TOTAL	Carbs Fat Protein Cals TOTAL	Carbs Fat Protein Cals TOTAL	Carbs Fat Protein Cals TOTAL
Tuesday	Carbs Fat Protein Cals TOTAL	Carbs Fat Protein Cals TOTAL	Carbs Fat Protein Cals TOTAL	Carbs Fat Protein Cals TOTAL	Carbs Fat Protein Cals TOTAL
Wednesday	Carbs Fat Protein Cals TOTAL	Carbs Fat Protein Cals TOTAL	Carbs Fat Protein Cals TOTAL	Carbs Fat Protein Cals TOTAL	Carbs Fat Protein Cals TOTAL
Thursday	Carbs Fat Protein Cals TOTAL	Carbs Fat Protein Cals TOTAL	Carbs Fat Protein Cals TOTAL	Carbs Fat Protein Cals TOTAL	Carbs Fat Protein Cals TOTAL
Friday	Carbs Fat Protein Cals TOTAL	Carbs Fat Protein Cals TOTAL	Carbs Fat Protein Cals TOTAL	Carbs Fat Protein Cals TOTAL	Carbs Fat Protein Cals TOTAL
Saturday	Carbs Fat Protein Cals TOTAL	Carbs Fat Protein Cals TOTAL	Carbs Fat Protein Cals TOTAL	Carbs Fat Protein Cals TOTAL	Carbs Fat Protein Cals TOTAL
Sunday	Carbs Fat Protein Cals TOTAL	Carbs Fat Protein Cals TOTAL	Carbs Fat Protein Cals TOTAL	Carbs Fat Protein Cals TOTAL	Carbs Fat Protein Cals TOTAL

Weekly Meal Planner

Week 2

	Breakfast	Lunch	Dinner	Snack	Other
Monday	Carbs Fat Protein Cals TOTAL	Carbs Fat Protein Cals TOTAL	Carbs Fat Protein Cals TOTAL	Carbs Fat Protein Cals TOTAL	Carbs Fat Protein Cals TOTAL
Tuesday	Carbs Fat Protein Cals TOTAL	Carbs Fat Protein Cals TOTAL	Carbs Fat Protein Cals TOTAL	Carbs Fat Protein Cals TOTAL	Carbs Fat Protein Cals TOTAL
Wednesday	Carbs Fat Protein Cals TOTAL	Carbs Fat Protein Cals TOTAL	Carbs Fat Protein Cals TOTAL	Carbs Fat Protein Cals TOTAL	Carbs Fat Protein Cals TOTAL
Thursday	Carbs Fat Protein Cals TOTAL	Carbs Fat Protein Cals TOTAL	Carbs Fat Protein Cals TOTAL	Carbs Fat Protein Cals TOTAL	Carbs Fat Protein Cals TOTAL
Friday	Carbs Fat Protein Cals TOTAL	Carbs Fat Protein Cals TOTAL	Carbs Fat Protein Cals TOTAL	Carbs Fat Protein Cals TOTAL	Carbs Fat Protein Cals TOTAL
Saturday	Carbs Fat Protein Cals TOTAL	Carbs Fat Protein Cals TOTAL	Carbs Fat Protein Cals TOTAL	Carbs Fat Protein Cals TOTAL	Carbs Fat Protein Cals TOTAL
Sunday	Carbs Fat Protein Cals TOTAL	Carbs Fat Protein Cals TOTAL	Carbs Fat Protein Cals TOTAL	Carbs Fat Protein Cals TOTAL	Carbs Fat Protein Cals TOTAL

Weekly Meal Planner

Week 3

	Breakfast	Lunch	Dinner	Snack	Other
Monday	Carbs Fat Protein Cals TOTAL	Carbs Fat Protein Cals TOTAL	Carbs Fat Protein Cals TOTAL	Carbs Fat Protein Cals TOTAL	Carbs Fat Protein Cals TOTAL
Tuesday	Carbs Fat Protein Cals TOTAL	Carbs Fat Protein Cals TOTAL	Carbs Fat Protein Cals TOTAL	Carbs Fat Protein Cals TOTAL	Carbs Fat Protein Cals TOTAL
Wednesday	Carbs Fat Protein Cals TOTAL	Carbs Fat Protein Cals TOTAL	Carbs Fat Protein Cals TOTAL	Carbs Fat Protein Cals TOTAL	Carbs Fat Protein Cals TOTAL
Thursday	Carbs Fat Protein Cals TOTAL	Carbs Fat Protein Cals TOTAL	Carbs Fat Protein Cals TOTAL	Carbs Fat Protein Cals TOTAL	Carbs Fat Protein Cals TOTAL
Friday	Carbs Fat Protein Cals TOTAL	Carbs Fat Protein Cals TOTAL	Carbs Fat Protein Cals TOTAL	Carbs Fat Protein Cals TOTAL	Carbs Fat Protein Cals TOTAL
Saturday	Carbs Fat Protein Cals TOTAL	Carbs Fat Protein Cals TOTAL	Carbs Fat Protein Cals TOTAL	Carbs Fat Protein Cals TOTAL	Carbs Fat Protein Cals TOTAL
Sunday	Carbs Fat Protein Cals TOTAL	Carbs Fat Protein Cals TOTAL	Carbs Fat Protein Cals TOTAL	Carbs Fat Protein Cals TOTAL	Carbs Fat Protein Cals TOTAL

Weekly Meal Planner

Week 4

	Breakfast	Lunch	Dinner	Snack	Other
Monday	Carbs Fat Protein Cals — TOTAL	Carbs Fat Protein Cals — TOTAL	Carbs Fat Protein Cals — TOTAL	Carbs Fat Protein Cals — TOTAL	Carbs Fat Protein Cals — TOTAL
Tuesday	Carbs Fat Protein Cals — TOTAL	Carbs Fat Protein Cals — TOTAL	Carbs Fat Protein Cals — TOTAL	Carbs Fat Protein Cals — TOTAL	Carbs Fat Protein Cals — TOTAL
Wednesday	Carbs Fat Protein Cals — TOTAL	Carbs Fat Protein Cals — TOTAL	Carbs Fat Protein Cals — TOTAL	Carbs Fat Protein Cals — TOTAL	Carbs Fat Protein Cals — TOTAL
Thursday	Carbs Fat Protein Cals — TOTAL	Carbs Fat Protein Cals — TOTAL	Carbs Fat Protein Cals — TOTAL	Carbs Fat Protein Cals — TOTAL	Carbs Fat Protein Cals — TOTAL
Friday	Carbs Fat Protein Cals — TOTAL	Carbs Fat Protein Cals — TOTAL	Carbs Fat Protein Cals — TOTAL	Carbs Fat Protein Cals — TOTAL	Carbs Fat Protein Cals — TOTAL
Saturday	Carbs Fat Protein Cals — TOTAL	Carbs Fat Protein Cals — TOTAL	Carbs Fat Protein Cals — TOTAL	Carbs Fat Protein Cals — TOTAL	Carbs Fat Protein Cals — TOTAL
Sunday	Carbs Fat Protein Cals — TOTAL	Carbs Fat Protein Cals — TOTAL	Carbs Fat Protein Cals — TOTAL	Carbs Fat Protein Cals — TOTAL	Carbs Fat Protein Cals — TOTAL

WEEK 1   MEDITERRANEAN *Meal* LOG BOOK

	BREAKFAST	LUNCH	DINNER	SNACKS
MONDAY				
TUESDAY				
WEDNESDAY				
THURSDAY				
FRIDAY				
SATURDAY				
SUNDAY				

WEEK 2 MEDITERRANEAN *Meal* LOG BOOK

	BREAKFAST	LUNCH	DINNER	SNACKS
MONDAY				
TUESDAY				
WEDNESDAY				
THURSDAY				
FRIDAY				
SATURDAY				
SUNDAY				

WEEK 3   MEDITERRANEAN *Meal* LOG BOOK

	BREAKFAST	LUNCH	DINNER	SNACKS
MONDAY				
TUESDAY				
WEDNESDAY				
THURSDAY				
FRIDAY				
SATURDAY				
SUNDAY				
	BREAKFAST	LUNCH	DINNER	SNACKS

WEEK 4   MEDITERRANEAN *Meal* LOG BOOK

	BREAKFAST	LUNCH	DINNER	SNACKS
MONDAY				
TUESDAY				
WEDNESDAY				
THURSDAY				
FRIDAY				
SATURDAY				
SUNDAY				

Low Carb Grocery Ideas

FRESH PRODUCE

☐ Asparagus	☐ Cauliflower	☐ Onions
☐ Avocado	☐ Celery	☐ Radishes
☐ Bell Peppers	☐ Cucumber	☐ Salad Mix
☐ Berries	☐ Eggplant	☐ Squash
☐ Broccoli	☐ Fennel	☐ Tomatoes
☐ Brussel Sprouts	☐ Garlic	☐ Bok Choi
☐ Cabbage	☐ Green Beans	☐ Chives
☐ Carrots	☐ Mushrooms	☐ Spinach

MEAT AND SEAFOOD

☐ Bacon	☐ Lamb	☐ Fish
☐ Beef	☐ Pork	☐ Crab
☐ Bison	☐ Rotisserie Chicken	☐ Lobster
☐ Chicken	☐ Sausage	☐ Scallops
☐ Deli meat	☐ Turkey	☐ Shrimp
☐ Ground Beef / Ground Turkey	☐ Oyster	☐ Mussels

DAIRY PRODUCTS

☐ Butter	☐ Eggs	☐ Sour Cream
☐ Cheese	☐ Greek Yogurt, full fat	☐ Ghee
☐ Cream Cheese	☐ Heavy Whipping Cream	☐ Mayo

PANTRY ITEMS

☐ Avocado oil	☐ Tea/Coffee	☐ Moon Cheese
☐ Beef Jerky	☐ Pork Rinds	☐ Low Carb Protein Bars
☐ Bone Broth	☐ Mayonnaise	☐ All Natural Peanut Butter
☐ Tuna, Salmon (canned)	☐ Low Carb Salad Dressing	☐ Stevia
☐ Coconut Butter	☐ Olive oil, extra virgin	☐ Almonds
☐ Coconut Oil	☐ Olives	☐ Spices
☐ Almond Milk	☐ Sweeteners	☐ Almond Flour

FROZEN / OTHER

☐	☐	☐
☐	☐	☐
☐	☐	☐
☐	☐	☐

Low Carb Shopping List — WEEK 1

FRESH PRODUCE

MEAT AND SEAFOOD

DAIRY PRODUCTS

PANTRY ITEMS

FROZEN / OTHER

Low Carb Shopping List — WEEK 2

FRESH PRODUCE

MEAT AND SEAFOOD

DAIRY PRODUCTS

PANTRY ITEMS

FROZEN / OTHER

Low Carb Shopping List — WEEK 3

FRESH PRODUCE

MEAT AND SEAFOOD

DAIRY PRODUCTS

PANTRY ITEMS

FROZEN / OTHER

Low Carb Shopping List

WEEK 4

FRESH PRODUCE

MEAT AND SEAFOOD

DAIRY PRODUCTS

PANTRY ITEMS

FROZEN / OTHER

Mediterranean *Recipe #1*

RECIPE NAME:
_____

Seafood	Low Carb	Paleo	Vegetarian	Vegan	Dairy Free	Gluten Free
☐	☐	☐	☐	☐	☐	☐

QTY	INGREDIENTS

RECIPE INSTRUCTIONS

NOTES & RECIPE REVIEW

Serves	
Prep Time	
Cook Time	
Tools	
Temp	

Total	Carbs	Fat	Protein	Cals

Mediterranean *Recipe #2*

RECIPE NAME:
_____

☐ Seafood ☐ Low Carb ☐ Paleo ☐ Vegetarian ☐ Vegan ☐ Dairy Free ☐ Gluten Free

QTY	INGREDIENTS

RECIPE INSTRUCTIONS

NOTES & RECIPE REVIEW

Serves	
Prep Time	
Cook Time	
Tools	
Temp	

Total	Carbs	Fat	Protein	Cals

Mediterranean *Recipe #3*

RECIPE NAME:
_____

	Seafood	Low Carb	Paleo	Vegetarian	Vegan	Dairy Free	Gluten Free
	☐	☐	☐	☐	☐	☐	☐

QTY	INGREDIENTS	RECIPE INSTRUCTIONS

NOTES & RECIPE REVIEW

Serves	
Prep Time	
Cook Time	
Tools	
Temp	

Total	Carbs	Fat	Protein	Cals

Mediterranean *Recipe #4*

RECIPE NAME:

Seafood ☐ Low Carb ☐ Paleo ☐ Vegetarian ☐ Vegan ☐ Dairy Free ☐ Gluten Free ☐

QTY	INGREDIENTS

RECIPE INSTRUCTIONS

NOTES & RECIPE REVIEW

Serves	
Prep Time	
Cook Time	
Tools	
Temp	

Total	Carbs	Fat	Protein	Cals

Mediterranean *Recipe #5*

RECIPE NAME:
_____

Seafood	Low Carb	Paleo	Vegetarian	Vegan	Dairy Free	Gluten Free
☐	☐	☐	☐	☐	☐	☐

QTY	INGREDIENTS	RECIPE INSTRUCTIONS

NOTES & RECIPE REVIEW

Serves	
Prep Time	
Cook Time	
Tools	
Temp	

Total	Carbs	Fat	Protein	Cals

Mediterranean *Recipe #6*

RECIPE NAME:
_____

| Seafood | Low Carb | Paleo | Vegetarian | Vegan | Dairy Free | Gluten Free |
| ☐ | ☐ | ☐ | ☐ | ☐ | ☐ | ☐ |

QTY	INGREDIENTS	RECIPE INSTRUCTIONS

NOTES & RECIPE REVIEW

Serves	
Prep Time	
Cook Time	
Tools	
Temp	

Total	Carbs	Fat	Protein	Cals

Mediterranean *Recipe #7*

RECIPE NAME:

☐ Seafood ☐ Low Carb ☐ Paleo ☐ Vegetarian ☐ Vegan ☐ Dairy Free ☐ Gluten Free

QTY	INGREDIENTS

RECIPE INSTRUCTIONS

NOTES & RECIPE REVIEW

Serves	
Prep Time	
Cook Time	
Tools	
Temp	

Total	Carbs	Fat	Protein	Cals

Mediterranean *Recipe #8*

RECIPE NAME:

Seafood ☐   Low Carb ☐   Paleo ☐   Vegetarian ☐   Vegan ☐   Dairy Free ☐   Gluten Free ☐

QTY	INGREDIENTS

RECIPE INSTRUCTIONS

NOTES & RECIPE REVIEW

Serves	
Prep Time	
Cook Time	
Tools	
Temp	

Total	Carbs	Fat	Protein	Cals

Mediterranean *Recipe #9*

RECIPE NAME:

☐ Seafood ☐ Low Carb ☐ Paleo ☐ Vegetarian ☐ Vegan ☐ Dairy Free ☐ Gluten Free

QTY	INGREDIENTS

RECIPE INSTRUCTIONS

NOTES & RECIPE REVIEW

Serves	
Prep Time	
Cook Time	
Tools	
Temp	

Total	Carbs	Fat	Protein	Cals

Mediterranean *Recipe #10*

RECIPE NAME:

	Seafood	Low Carb	Paleo	Vegetarian	Vegan	Dairy Free	Gluten Free
	☐	☐	☐	☐	☐	☐	☐

QTY	INGREDIENTS	RECIPE INSTRUCTIONS

NOTES & RECIPE REVIEW

Serves	
Prep Time	
Cook Time	
Tools	
Temp	

Total	Carbs	Fat	Protein	Cals

WEIGHT LOSS *Journal*

MONDAY

TUESDAY

WEDNESDAY

THURSDAY

FRIDAY

SATURDAY

SUNDAY

WEEK OF:

DATE	WEIGHT LOSS ACTION PLAN

NOTES

WEIGHT LOSS *Journal*

MONDAY

TUESDAY

WEDNESDAY

THURSDAY

FRIDAY

SATURDAY

SUNDAY

WEEK OF:

DATE	WEIGHT LOSS ACTION PLAN

NOTES

WEIGHT LOSS *Journal*

MONDAY

TUESDAY

WEDNESDAY

THURSDAY

FRIDAY

SATURDAY

SUNDAY

WEEK OF:

DATE	WEIGHT LOSS ACTION PLAN

NOTES

WEIGHT LOSS *Journal*

MONDAY

TUESDAY

WEDNESDAY

THURSDAY

FRIDAY

SATURDAY

SUNDAY

WEEK OF:

DATE	WEIGHT LOSS ACTION PLAN

NOTES

GOALS & *Accomplishments*

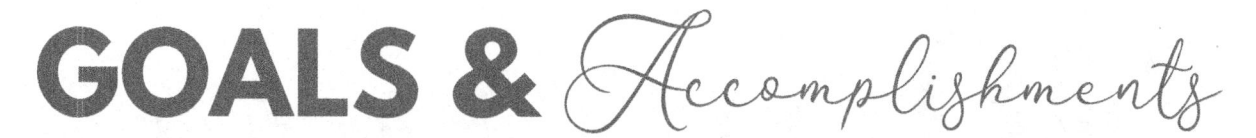

MONTH   JAN   FEB   MAR   APR   MAY   JUN   JUL   AUG   SEP   OCT   NOV   DEC

THIS MONTH'S GOALS

ACTION PLAN

M T W T F S S

NOTES:

WEEKLY GOALS

M
T
W
T
F
S
S

THOUGHTS

MEALS:	BREAKFAST	LUNCH	DINNER	SNACKS
M				
T				
W				
T				
F				
S				
S				

30 Days of Med

STARTING WEIGHT:

DAY 30 WEIGHT:

| 1 | 2 | 3 | 4 | 5 | 6 | 7 | 8 | 9 | 10 |

LBS LOST:
INCHES LOST:

| 11 | 12 | 13 | 14 | 15 | 16 | 17 | 18 | 19 | 20 |

LBS LOST:
INCHES LOST:

| 21 | 22 | 23 | 24 | 25 | 26 | 27 | 28 | 29 | 30 |

LBS LOST:
INCHES LOST:

TOTAL WEIGHT LOST:

TOTAL INCHES LOST:

NOTES:

PERSONAL ACCOMPLISHMENTS:

THOUGHTS & REFLECTIONS:

60 Days of MED

STARTING WEIGHT: **DAY 60 WEIGHT:**

1	2	3	4	5	6	7	8	9	10	**LBS LOST:** **INCHES LOST:**
11	12	13	14	15	16	17	18	19	20	**LBS LOST:** **INCHES LOST:**
21	22	23	24	25	26	27	28	29	30	**LBS LOST:** **INCHES LOST:**
31	32	33	34	35	36	37	38	39	40	**LBS LOST:** **INCHES LOST:**
41	42	43	44	45	46	47	48	49	50	**LBS LOST:** **INCHES LOST:**
51	52	53	54	55	56	57	58	59	60	**LBS LOST:** **INCHES LOST:**

TOTAL WEIGHT LOST: **TOTAL INCHES LOST:**

NOTES & REFLECTIONS:

100 Days of Med

STARTING WEIGHT:

DAY 100 WEIGHT:

1	2	3	4	5	6	7	8	9	10	**LBS LOST:** **INCHES LOST:**
11	12	13	14	15	16	17	18	19	20	**LBS LOST:** **INCHES LOST:**
21	22	23	24	25	26	27	28	29	30	**LBS LOST:** **INCHES LOST:**
31	32	33	34	35	36	37	38	39	40	**LBS LOST:** **INCHES LOST:**
41	42	43	44	45	46	47	48	49	50	**LBS LOST:** **INCHES LOST:**
51	52	53	54	55	56	57	58	59	60	**LBS LOST:** **INCHES LOST:**
61	62	63	64	65	66	67	68	69	70	**LBS LOST:** **INCHES LOST:**
71	72	73	74	75	76	77	78	79	80	**LBS LOST:** **INCHES LOST:**
81	82	83	84	85	86	87	88	89	90	**LBS LOST:** **INCHES LOST:**
91	92	93	94	95	96	97	98	99	100	**LBS LOST:** **INCHES LOST:**

TOTAL WEIGHT LOST:

TOTAL INCHES LOST:

NOTES & REFLECTIONS:

Notes

Notes

Notes

Notes

Notes

Notes

Notes

Notes

Made in the USA
Monee, IL
20 January 2025